Right Food Right Weight

Use your slow metabolism to lose weight

By Bradford Chase, MPAS

About the Author

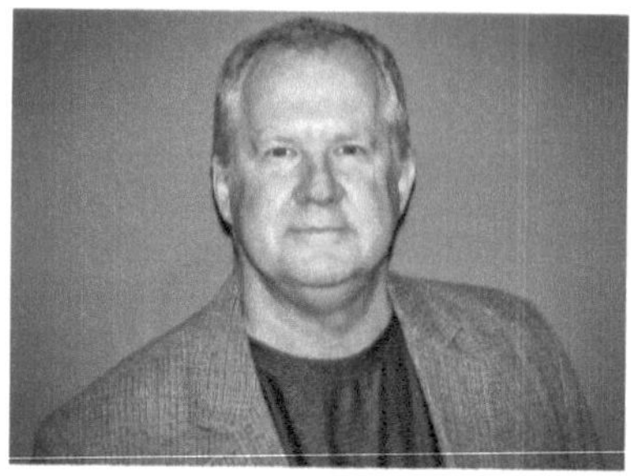

Brad Chase has more than 30 years of experience in healthcare. He graduated with honors from Wake Forest University School of Medicine in North Carolina as a Physician Assistant. Although his training focused on Internal Medicine, he worked for many years in bariatric medicine and specialized in helping patients struggling with the difficulties of weight loss. He believes in the importance of treating the mind, body, and spirit for total wellness. He has traveled as a national speaker for the American Academy of Physician Assistants, and lectured on topics of both health and leadership.

Cover Photo By

Pablo Merchán Montes

Table Of Contents

Before You Start

It is always important to work with your own healthcare provider when starting any weight loss program. They are much more familiar with your personal health history and are the best source for identifying things that may help you lose weight, and things that may not be appropriate for your current health status. For example, if you have a history of kidney stones or other kidney disease, you need to be careful about the amount of protein in your diet.

Always check with your health care provider before starting any new exercise program for the same reasons.

Always make your health care provider aware of any natural vitamins and supplements you are interested in trying. Even those that are classified as "natural" can still interact with certain prescription medications. It is important that you don't assume something is safe just because you bought it at a "Health Food" store or a local vitamin shop.

The information provided is based on personal, clinical, and professional experience as well as current scientific research information obtained from multiple public sources.

Every journey we take starts with our next step. Only tomorrow will tell how successful that journey will be, and we must always remember:

Failing to do anything is still failing...

We all know when we eat better, we feel better; about ourselves and about our health.

Medical research shows us when we focus on better nutrition; we improve our chances for longevity.

Even more exciting; it is a proven fact that successfully reaching weight and nutrition goals makes us much more likely to be successful in other areas of our life as well[1].

Weight loss is a sensitive subject for all of us. It's easy to gain weight and very difficult to lose it. If it was easy, we'd never need to read a book like this or worry about what we eat.

So we agree this is difficult. There is no easy way through the process.

Let's start by going through a refresher course in basic nutrition and then talk about how this information affects the calories we eat.

Then we discuss metabolism and how it works for or against us in losing weight.

Finally, I'll provide you with a new type of eating program that gives you the power to harness your own metabolism work for you.

This book is not directed toward any specific diet choice or food belief system.

If you are a vegan, and vegetarian, or a meat eater, the information you find in this book will work in helping to improve your diet and nutrition education.

NUTRITION

Exploring nutrition in detail is extensive course by itself, taking years to master. This book isn't an in-depth look into nutrition. Our review is focused on understanding the science behind nutrition to create better daily food choices and know how they impact our health, weight control, and well-being.

Specifically, we need to understand how our body processes carbohydrates, fats, and protein and what that means in terms of healthy weight loss and healthy weight control.

Our discussion begins with Energy Production.

In the simplest terms of how we gain and lose weight, we've probably all heard the statement, "burn more calories than you take in and you will lose weight."

While this sounds like a simple concept, it is not. What is more frustrating is the manner in which is implies those of us who struggle with losing weight are just too lazy to burn more calories than we eat.

We know that idea is just not true.

The idea behind the statement is true, however. If we continue to eat more calories than our body uses as fuel, our body will store some of those calories to use in the future if needed.

In most cases, those calories get stored as fat.

If we constantly over eat the *wrong-type of calories*, then we constantly give our body the ability to keep storing more and more unneeded calories as fat, and we gain weight.

The struggle with losing the fat is based on how our body burns calories; it doesn't go after those stored fat cells first.

This a very simplistic description of why we feel like we gain weight easily and it become so difficult to lose it.

Our goal, then become trying to ***work with our body***, using our knowledge of how it stores and burns calories in a way that doesn't require us to significantly increase our ability to exercise and still target some of those fat stores by getting our current metabolism to burn the stored calories first.

ENERGY PRODUCTION

Let's look at how our body processes what we eat and turns it into the energy we need to function. This process is the backbone of learning how to what we eat becomes energy that fuels our systems or stored fat that causes weight gain.

We will look at three basic energy sources that our body can utilize; what they consist of, and how our body typically processes them throughout the day.

CARBOHYDRATES

Carbohydrates are the most basic form of energy and two type of carbohydrates are the first choice that our body utilizes for energy.

For our purposes, there are three types of carbohydrates we need to consider:

    1) Simple sugars or simple carbohydrates (one of which is glucose)
    2) Complex carbohydrates or Starches
    3) Fiber

Simple Carbohydrates

When our body needs quick energy the first thing it looks for are simple carbohydrates.

Simple carbohydrates are sugars made up of just one or two sugar molecules. They are very easily digested, can be used up quickly in the body for energy and include things such as table sugar, brown sugar, honey, fruit drinks, sodas, candy, etc.

Simple sugars are detrimental to our health when consumed in larger quantities than our current activity level requires and one of the worst things to eat in excess if your activity level does not dictate a regular need for quick and easy energy.

For many people, simple sugars are the number one cause of excess weight gain because they are hidden in a number of foods typically consumed in large quantities such as carbonated beverages (non-diet soda!) and sweetened foods with small serving sizes but <u>huge</u> amounts of simple sugar (donuts, breakfast cereal, snack cakes, candy bars, etc).

Complex Carbohydrates

When simple sugars join together and form longer chains these molecules become complex carbohydrates, also known as starches.

Because these molecules are more complex they typically require a few additional steps when processed in our body for energy.

Most of our healthier foods in the carbohydrate category contain complex carbohydrates or starches rather than simple sugars. It is important to remember, however, that there are some complex carbohydrates that are no better for you from a health standpoint than simple sugars. The key is how easily our body can break down a complex carbohydrate into a simple sugar. The easier the breakdown, the worse the food is from a nutritional viewpoint.

Examples of food sources complex carbohydrates include starchy vegetables such as potatoes, sweet potatoes, corn, etc.

On the healthier side green vegetables, whole grains, beans, lentils, and peas also contain complex carbohydrates but are much better for you from a nutritional standpoint than the starchy vegetables. These typically do not breakdown to simple sugars as easily and they contain a very healthy carbohydrate; Fiber.

Fiber

Fiber is also a complex carbohydrate, but it plays a very positive role in assisting to improve our health.

The body cannot digest fiber. It cannot be broken down into sugar molecules and instead passes through the body undigested.

Fiber does help to regulate the body's use of sugars as well as provides "bulk" to our meals and helps to control hunger. As you can imagine this plays an important part in basic nutrition as well as assist with weight control.

There are two types of fiber:

– **Soluble fiber**: soluble fiber dissolves in water and plays a part in glucose and cholesterol control in our bodies. Some of the foods that are high in soluble fiber includes; beans, lentils, nuts, and some fruits.

– **Insoluble fiber**: insoluble fiber is just that, fiber that does not dissolve in water. It can provide bulk to our digestive track which helps move food and helps to prevent constipation. A few of the foods that are high in insoluble fiber include wheat, whole grains, brown rice, carrots, and some beans.

INSULIN

Insulin is a hormone, not a carbohydrate, but I want to mention it here because of its role in our body. Most people only think of insulin as it relates to the disease of diabetes. The truth is, insulin is a key component of how our body processes carbohydrates.

Insulin is created in our pancreas, an organ located just adjacent and behind the stomach. The primary purpose of insulin is its role in directing muscle, fat and the liver to use glucose as our primary fuel.

Insulin lets carbohydrates we eat get used for energy immediately. In addition, insulin directs the muscles and liver to store extra carbohydrate as glycogen.

Glycogen is made up of combined glucose molecules similar to plant starches. Limited amounts of glycogen can be made since glycogen is meant to be a short term not a long term energy reserve.

People with Type 1 Diabetes have a pancreas that produces very little or no insulin so they need to inject insulin to properly utilize energy from foods they eat. For many type 1 diabetics, they developed the disease very early in life, and typically developed juvenile diabetes. Some adults lose the ability to produce insulin due to disease or injury and develop Type 1 Diabetes later in life.

People with Type 2 Diabetes are usually adults who have a functioning pancreas, but for some reason it no longer produces enough insulin to manage the carbohydrates they eat; either through a reduction in insulin production or their body tissues are now resistant to the normal levels of insulin production their pancreas is able to produce and so blood sugar levels are no longer controlled without medications.

Many overweight adults (and now some unfortunate significantly overweight children) lose the ability to process the insulin their body produces because of the resistance developed as a result of excess fat in their system. Too much fat in the blood stream increases tiny fat droplets inside muscle cells. This "gums up" the ability for insulin to let muscles cells properly use glucose. This is known as Insulin Resistance. Type 2 Diabetics must take medications that help to encourage muscles cells to use insulin in spite of the intramuscular fat droplets, or increase the amount of insulin through shots.

Type 2 Diabetes was once thought to be irreversible. We are now learning that for some obese adults with the disease, losing weight and eating better causes their body to once again utilized insulin they make and the disease is reversed as long as they maintain a healthy weight.

UNDERSTANDING WHY CARBS CAUSE WEIGHT GAIN

Our ability to store carbohydrates in the liver and muscle as glycogen is limited, so we need another means of storing excessive diet carbohydrate energy.

To do this, our liver and fat tissue converts some of the extra glucose to fat in the form of triglycerides. The fat made in our fat cells is stored within those cells. The triglycerides made in the liver are transported by the blood to fat cells and to a lesser degree other tissue such as muscle, breast tissue, etc.

We know our ability to convert excessive carbohydrate to fat is not a very efficient process. The body prefers to use excessive carbohydrates for energy and can do that much more efficiently than turning them into body fat.

So why does consuming excessive carbohydrates make us fat?

When we eat a diet high in excessive carbohydrates, our body will stop burning stored fat as energy. We are providing our body with the energy source it needs immediately in the carbohydrates we are eating.

In addition, any fat we eat while the body is burning carbohydrates is just stored for later, adding to our already increasing fat content.

The increased fat in the bloodstream makes the body's need for insulin greater to use the carbohydrates we are eating as energy. This exacerbates the insulin resistance problem that creates Type 2 Diabetes.

This situation tends to happen more when people eat a larger number of carbohydrate and fat calories during the day then they need for energy based on their activity levels, *especially* when those calories are consumed as simple carbohydrates (high sugar foods and drinks).

Because of the process discussed above, this is also a greater problem for people who have type 2 diabetes or have developed a level of insulin resistance; sometimes referred to as pre-diabetes.

GLYCEMIC INDEX and GLYCEMIC LOAD

Another important aspect of carbohydrates we need to consider is Glycemic Index and Glycemic Load.

Understanding the glycemic impact can have a direct impact on your health:

- Eating many high-glycemic-index foods – which cause powerful spikes in blood sugar and exacerbate insulin resistance – can lead to an increased risk for type 2 diabetes, heart disease, and becoming overweight.
- There are studies linking high-glycemic diets to age-related macular degeneration, infertility, and colorectal cancer.
- Foods with a low glycemic index have been shown to help control type 2 diabetes and improve weight loss.

Glycemic Index

The glycemic index ranks carbohydrates on a scale from 0 to 100 based on how quickly and how much they raise blood sugar levels after eating. Foods with a high glycemic index, like white bread, are rapidly digested and cause substantial changes quickly in blood sugar. Foods with a low glycemic index, like whole oats, are digested more slowly, prompting a more gradual rise in blood sugar.

Glycemic Load

One thing that a food's glycemic index does not tell us is how much digestible carbohydrate – the total amount of carbohydrates excluding fiber – it delivers. That's why researchers developed a related way to classify foods that takes into account both the amount of carbohydrate in the food in relation to its impact on blood sugar levels. This measure is called the glycemic load.

A food's glycemic load is determined by multiplying its glycemic index by the amount of carbohydrate the food contains. In general, a glycemic load of 20 or more is high, 11 to 19 is medium, and 10 or under is low.

Glycemic loads are important to determine if what we eat increases our chance of certain diseases based on our carbohydrate intake.

There was a large meta-analysis of 24 prospective cohort studies which concluded that people who consumed lower-glycemic load diets were at a lower risk of developing type 2 diabetes[2].

Those who ate a diet of higher-glycemic load foods were are a much greater risk for developing type 2 diabetes and heart problems. A different but similar study concluded that higher-glycemic load diets were also associated with an increased risk for heart attacks as well.

To give you an idea about how foods compare, here is a listing of low, medium, and high glycemic load foods.

The idea is to try to focus on daily diets that have a larger amount of low glycemic load foods, allows limited medium glycemic load foods and try's to avoid the high glycemic load foods as much as practical.

EXAMPLES OF GLYCEMIC LOADS IN FOOD

Low glycemic load (10 or under)

- Bran cereals
- Apple
- Orange
- Kidney beans
- Black beans
- Lentils
- Wheat tortilla
- Skim milk
- Cashews
- Peanuts
- Carrots

Medium glycemic load (11-19)

- Pearled barley
- Brown rice
- Oatmeal
- Bulgur
- Rice cakes
- Whole grain breads
- Whole-grain pasta

High glycemic load (20+)

- Baked potato
- French fries
- Refined breakfast cereal
- Sugar-sweetened beverages
- Candy bars
- Couscous
- White basmati rice
- White-flour pasta

FATS

Just like all carbohydrates are not the same; all fats are not the same either and while there are many, we are going to limit our discussion for the purposes of this book to:

1. Saturated Fats
2. Trans-Fats
3. Unsaturated Fats
   - Monounsaturated fats
   - Polyunsaturated fats
   - Omega-3 fatty acids

Fat is an important part of our diet and is required for optimum health.

With that said, it is important that we eat the correct types of fats and limit our intake to correct amounts.

The term "saturated" and "unsaturated" is due to the chemical makeup of the fats and how hydrogen and carbon atoms are part of that make up.

For our purposes it's not as important to know why they are called by these two terms, but more important to know what each type of fat is in relation to our discussion of nutrition.

THE FATS WE TEND TO THINK OF AS HARMFUL

Saturated Fats

As a rule, saturated fats are solid at room temperature.

Not all saturated fats come from animal sources and they do not all have cholesterol in them, but they all can have some impact on our own cholesterol production. It is important to make that distinction when looking at fats in our diet.

While we know that saturated fats can lead to increased LDL cholesterol in our bodies, we should _not_ make a general statement that saturated fat is "bad".

Coconut oil and palm oil are two vegetable oils that are made up primarily of saturated fats but may offer limited benefits to our nutritional intake when eaten in moderation, and add no dietary cholesterol to our diets.

The key is –moderation — due to the know ties between saturated fat and heart disease. The confusion comes because some studies show the type of saturated fats found in coconut and palm oils can help lower triglycerides and help to raise HDL cholesterol in our bodies.

Coconut oil is not a health food, contrary to popular belief. It may contain some beneficial properties, but due to the very high levels of saturated fats it must be consumed in moderation or it becomes unhealthy.

Fats that contain cholesterol only come from things with livers; where cholesterol is made. So animal fats can be saturated and contain cholesterol, but vegetable fats can also be saturated, but will not contain any cholesterol.

[To be scientifically correct, plants can have a type of cholesterol called phytosterols, which are toxic to humans, so the intestines are designed not to absorb them.]

If we are someone that needs to limit the intake of dietary cholesterol than we need to make certain that we move away from saturated fats, especially fats that come from animal sources

Trans Fats

Trans fats are only found in small amount naturally in some foods. When we find trans fats in our diet, it likely comes from processed foods that are otherwise not a healthy choice.

Most of our current exposure to trans fats comes from hydrogenation.

This is a chemical process in which hydrogen is added to liquid oils to turn them into a solid form.

Partially hydrogenated fat molecules have trans fats, and may be the worst type of fat we consume.

It is important not to confuse man-made trans fats with those that occur naturally in some foods. Only chemically altered trans fats have been shown to increase cholesterol levels, which can lead to a host of cardiovascular problems.

These fats used to be wide spread in fast foods, but are at least somewhat less prevalent today; however you still need to be cautious about eating any fried foods in restaurants, margarines, anything with vegetable shortening in it (pie crusts, biscuits, etc), to avoid trans fats. Always look at the labels.

Our goal will be to avoid all man-made trans fats in all our daily diet choices

THE FATS WE TEND TO THINK OF AS MORE HEALTHFUL

Unsaturated Fats

Foods made up mostly of monounsaturated and polyunsaturated fats are liquid at room temperature.

When we add fat to our diet in any form, these are the fats we want to focus on as a more health choice in most respects.

Monounsaturated fats

This is a type of fat found in a variety of foods and oils.

Studies show that eating food high in monounsaturated fats can improve our cholesterol levels[3].

Research also shows that these fats may offer some benefit in controlling insulin levels and blood sugar levels[4].

Examples of oils rich in monounsaturated fat include olive, peanut, canola, sunflower and sesame. Examples of nuts include almonds, peanuts, cashews, Brazil nuts, hazelnuts, macadamia nuts, pecans, and pistachios. Vegetables include avocados, and black and green olives.

Polyunsaturated fats

This is a type of fat found mostly in plant-based foods and oils.

Evidence shows that eating foods rich in polyunsaturated fats improves our blood cholesterol levels[3].

This may also decrease our risk of heart disease.

There are a few studies that indicate polyunsaturated fats may also help decrease the risk of type 2 diabetes[4].

Examples of oils rich in polyunsaturated fats include flaxseed, walnut, canola and soybean oil. Cold water or "fatty" Fish are also a good source of these healthier fats.

Omega – 3 Fatty Acids

This is actually a subcategory of polyunsaturated fat, but always raises a lot of questions.

Omega-3 fatty acids, found in some types of fatty fish, appear to decrease the risk of coronary artery disease. It may also protect against irregular heartbeats and help lower blood pressure levels.

When looking at sources for Omega-3 fatty acids, although there are plant sources, the body doesn't convert these easily or use them as well as omega-3 from fish. Flaxseed oil is probably the best source from plants.

Why Too Much Fat Causes Us to Gain Weight

Fat is our body's second favorite source of energy.

Because of the way fat is processed in our body, the fat we eat tends to go directly into storage and the fat already stored is used first for energy.

When we consume more fat than our body burns for energy during the day, we gain weight.

As previously mentions, this is worse when we eat a lot of carbohydrates and sugars along with fat.

The body will tend to use the sugars for energy first, so the dietary fat just gets stored along with the body fat that is now no longer being burned, adding to our weight gain.

A diet high in fat is unhealthy. A diet high in both fat and sugar is a much faster way to gain weight than just fat or just sugar alone.

Consider this point very closely when looking at food choices. High fat meals found at fast food restaurants combined with high sugar drinks found at fast food restaurants is the easiest way to ensure that you gain weight quickly.

You pay for convenience with weight gain, so you need to consider what your priorities are every time you make a food choice. You can't have it both ways.

PROTEINS

Proteins are made up from of combinations of amino acids.

There are 20 different amino acids that join together to make all types of protein.

We have the ability to make some of these amino acids in our body; these are called non-essential amino acids because we it is no essential to get them in our diet.

More importantly, there are 9 amino acids that we can't make ourselves, so these are called as *essential* amino acids.

Proper nutrition requires we include the essential amino acids in our diet and in the correct proportions.

You may also hear the terms compete and incomplete protein source. It is important to make certain that the proteins we do eat are complete in the required amino acids in order to be considered for providing the appropriate nutritional resources that our bodies need.

Complete Proteins

Complete protein sources are capable of supplying all of the 9 different essential amino acids and providing them in the correct proportions. If the protein lacks even one of the essential amino acids then it cannot be considered complete.

In general complete proteins include all animal and fish proteins. This includes meats and fish, poultry, cheese, eggs, yogurt, milk, etc.

Plants such as soy, quinoa, chia, and hemp contain all 9 of the essential amino acids.

The biggest difference in meat or dairy sources of protein and plant sources of protein is the total amount of protein available in a normal serving.

Animal and dairy products typically have more protein per serving than plant sources.

Incomplete Proteins

Incomplete proteins are any protein lacking one or more essential amino acid or don't have correct proportions of these essential amino acids. They are also called partial proteins. In general, incomplete proteins come from plant sources. Examples of incomplete proteins include grains, nuts, beans, seeds, peas, corn, etc.

It's not critical we get every essential amino acid every time we eat; we just need to be certain we get an appropriate amount of the essential amino acids every day in our normal diet.

Complimentary Proteins

It is possible to combine incomplete proteins to create complete proteins.

The amino acids missing from one type of food can be compensated by adding a protein containing the missing amino acid in another type of food. When eaten together in the same meal this combination provides us will all essential amino acids. When combined together like this, proteins are considered complementary. Examples of complementary proteins would include; grains with legumes, nuts with legumes, etc.

With the large variety of protein sources available combined with the multiple resources for creative menu planning available on the Internet, it is easy to get the necessary amounts of protein with essential amino acids in any type of diet. This includes vegetarian and vegan options.

What about Gluten?

Gluten is the main protein complex in wheat, barley, rye, and triticale (a cross between wheat and rye).

Due to the significant publicity surrounding gluten, gluten free diets, and perceived side effects from eating gluten, this can be a polarizing subject.

But I think we need to talk about it.

I base my information on scientific data, research studies, and actual patient experience working for years in Internal Medicine. I do not give any credit to anecdotal information from the internet, celebrities, or TV personalities trying to jump on the gluten bandwagon and sell a new program.

With money being spent on gluten free products and the number of gluten free products that are now available, it's important to make sure that we understand exactly what gluten is and if eating gluten is always an issue.
The quick and easy answer is; if you are someone diagnosed by a medical professional with celiac disease, then gluten is definitely something you have to avoid.

If you do not have celiac disease or a true gluten allergy, then gluten is not your enemy as many would like to believe.

In fact, following a strictly gluten free diet when no medical condition exists can actually create new health problems for you[5].

While gluten itself doesn't offer special nutritional benefits the potential problems with gluten free diets for people who do not have a gluten allergy are these;

1. Many whole grains that contain gluten are rich in vitamins and minerals, such as B vitamins and iron, as well as fiber. Removing whole grains can lead to vitamin and mineral deficiencies and associated health problems
2. Many gluten free products are far from healthy and are more likely to contain saturated fats, cholesterol, and high calorie content
3. Many gluten free products are comprised of simple sugars and unhealthy carbohydrates that can cause blood sugar concerns and actually cause weight gain

In addition, gluten free products tend to be more expensive than gluten containing similar products.

While there are individuals without any gluten sensitivity reporting they've lost weight and feel better after removing gluten from their diets, many admit they are eating more fresh vegetables, more lean meats, and paying more attention to the types of food they eat.

All of these dietary adjustments may be responsible for their improved feeling of well-being and weight loss as any impact from just removing gluten.

There is no scientifically validated medical evidence that getting rid of gluten alone in your diet can cause weight loss or eating gluten will cause weight gain.

As a medical professional, I fully support making dietary changes that improve health and well being as long as these changes do not ultimately cause other health issues. Removing gluten from your diet is a personal choice when not medically necessary.

If you chose to remove gluten from your food, please be certain to ensure you follow a healthy choice of vitamin-rich foods to help prevent unexpected future health problems.

Why Too Much Protein Makes Us Fat

Protein has calories just like fat and carbohydrates. There are no fat-free proteins.

Remember, if we eat more calories than we burn during the day, our body may store those extra calories; they just don't disappear. For the purposes of weight gain, the body doesn't care where the extra calories come from.

The key is using protein calories to our advantage because it is the least favorite form of energy our body utilizes during normal activity. If we get most calories from protein, we force our body to first use up carbohydrates/sugars, and then fat for energy. This is why high protein diets typically are very effective for weight loss. It just isn't practical to always stick to a high protein diet. We need to find a balance that works with a normal lifestyle. Keep reading to find out how we make that happen.

FLUIDS

I want to take a minute to say something about fluid intake along with the three energy sources we just covered.

Water is crucial to good health and fluid intake is vital to allowing our bodies to properly process any energy sources we get from food we eat.

While we tend to focus on "drinking water" because it is the purest form of what our body needs, I tell my patients that "drinking fluids" is important. Realizing caffeinated or sweetened beverages can also have a negative impact on overall health goals, these beverages do count toward fluid intake requirements and so should not be considered outside of daily fluid needs. They just may not be the best choice for getting the fluids we need.

A number of recent studies found that drinking caffeinated beverages does not cause any concern with dehydration or counteract the hydration you receive from caffeinated beverages. The key is to drink something and avoid sugar.

Contrary to popular belief there is no standard amount of fluid adults must consume every. Our water needs depend on many factors including how healthy we are, how active we are, and where we live (environment plays a key role here as well).

Many health professionals recommend a minimum of "eight 8-ounce (approx. 237ml) glasses of fluid a day." This will supply us with about 1.9L of fluid and is a good place to start, but remember that your specific needs will vary.

Our bodies contain approximately 60% water by weight. Every one of our body systems depends on water to function.

Lack of water will lead to dehydration which is serious when severe, but even mild dehydration creates a feeling of fatigue and general malaise.

We lose water every day through normal breathing, perspiration, and bodily waste functions. It's important we constantly replenish the water supply we lose through these normal body functions.

Additional fluid intake is required if you exert yourself, live in an area where you perspire heavily, live at higher altitudes, or you have health issues that increase bodily waste functions such as vomiting, diarrhea or increased urination.

Can Too Much Water Be Harmful?

Yes. In general, too much of anything can be harmful.

More importantly, if you have certain medical conditions that cause you to retain fluids, such as heart failure or kidney disease, you may need to limit your fluid intake.

Drinking too much liquid can also result in an electrolyte imbalance. This is extremely rare if you follow common sense and the above recommendations.

If you are unsure of what your body requires, always consult your personal medical professional to find out exactly what your daily requirements may be.

As a general rule, if you rarely feel thirsty and your urine is colorless or light yellow it is likely your fluid intake is adequate.

It is recommended that you drink fluids with every meal as well as before, during, and after any exercise. Water or a low-calorie beverage is always best.

ONE OTHER HORMONE TO BE AWARE OF: LEPTIN

Leptin is a protein made in fat cells and circulates in the bloodstream. Leptin is the way your fat cells tell your brain your energy thermostat is set just right.

It helps control our hunger and our fat storage.

Leptin levels are set at a certain threshold, likely genetically set for each individual. When our leptin level is above our threshold, the brain senses we have adequate fat storage and energy requirement are being met.

Science believes when our leptin levels are above our set point, we burn energy at a normal rate, hunger and desire to eat are in a normal range and normal activity levels burn fat at a standard rate.

Because of how leptin works, dieting to lose weight causes a problem many of us are unaware of.

When we quickly cut back calories in our diet, we eat less and our fat cells lose some fat, which then decreases the amount of leptin produced.

Remember; when leptin is high, fat cells stop storing fat. When leptin is low, our brain feels we are starving and need to store more fat to survive.

Unfortunately, just like resistance to insulin can develop in people who are overweight, resistance to leptin can also develop, so while the fat cells keep growing and leptin production keeps increasing, the brain is not "seeing" these higher leptin levels. The brain continues to feel it needs more food to survive.

High triglycerides and high insulin levels also contribute to leptin resistance.

Think about this concept and the issues over years of dieting and gaining weight back. Your resistance to leptin works against future dieting attempts.

We need a way to combat feeling hungry and still working with the body to cause fat lose in a program that is a change in eating habits and not a "diet" that only works for short term.

I've developed one.

WEIGHT CONTROL, NUTRITION, AND METABOLISM

We've addressed basic nutrition, now let's look more in depth at why we gain weight, why we lose weight, and how our metabolism is involved these processes.

Weight Gain

Weight gain happens primarily for two reasons.

First, we consume excessive calories than required to function throughout the day. These excessive calories are stored for later use, typically as fat.

Second is hormonal, but I'm not talking about people who use "hormones" as an excuse for weight gain.

The vast majority of people who gain weight due to hormones do not start with a hormone problem. They develop hormone imbalances due to over-eating the wrong types of foods for years and create the problem themselves.

I know I sound abrupt, but we must admit the source and the struggle or we continue to pretend we can fix it with miracle cures and never conquer our weight problem.

You can get mad at me for being truthful with you, close this book now, ask for you money back, and stay overweight, or you can get motivated to make lifestyle changes what improve your long term health outlook.

There are people who have diseases and health problems causing weight gain unrelated to overeating.

The number of people with this problem is a very, very small part of the overweight population.

If your health care provider has looked and never found such an issue, the weight problem is not disease related.

They are easily diagnosed.

How does a hormone imbalance happen?

As previously discussed, large amounts of sugar in our diet (whether simple sugars, complex sugars, or converted starches) causes cells in our body to become resistant to the primary natural appetite suppressants of insulin and leptin; hormones found in our body.

When these natural appetite suppressants don't work, we are hungry more often and consume more calories which in turn create added fat stores and increase our resistance even more to our natural appetite suppressants.

As you can see, it can become a vicious cycle. <u>It's important to realize because of the hormonal fluctuations it is NOT weakness in willpower causing us to overeat</u>. It does take commitment to changing an unhealthy diet in order to impact our struggle to return our natural appetite suppressants to the proper function.

Weight Loss

Weight loss happens for number of reasons as well, all resulting in a loss of body mass.

Ideally we want this body mass to come from our fat stores however it is possible to lose muscle, water weight, and even bone density and all can contribute to a measurable weight loss.

It is a myth you can only lose fat by exercising.

In fact, in some cases exercise increases our demand for energy and thus increases our appetite and our caloric intake.

With the hormonal dysfunction that happens from our natural appetite suppressant resistance, we must use caution with exercising excessively as a primary means of causing weight loss.

For those of us overweight, we need to force our body to burn fat stores. This is not always in direct correlation to the number of calories we consume during the day. Specifically a low-calorie diet won't always produce significant or healthy weight loss in most normal adults.

Conventional wisdom assumes if we burned the same amount of calories we take in each day, our weight would be stable. Along those same lines of thinking , if we eat more calories than we burn, we gain weight and if we burn more calories than we eat, we lose weight.

While this sounds reasonable, it's based on a one-sided view of the laws of thermodynamics.

This law states matter can neither be destroyed nor created and indicates that if calories eaten equals calories burned there is no weight gain; continuing to look at this equation logically from a mathematical standpoint we could say that weight gain causes an increase in calories needed and weight loss causes a decrease in calories needed as well.

To understand caloric intake, weight loss, and weight gain, we need to approach this differently.

I want to look at this based on types of energy we use in our body, the diet that supplies the energy we use, and the importance of differentiating the energy types we eat for everyday function.

In doing this we don't discount the law of thermodynamics but instead refrain from misrepresenting the impact it has on our concept of weight gain or weight loss.

Most importantly remember; if you eat more calories than your body needs to function throughout the day you will gain weight.

You cannot overeat regularly and expect to maintain a healthy weight, and you cannot overeat and expect to lose weight.

We will focus on overcoming the resistance we've developed to our natural appetite suppressants of insulin and leptin, and developing a diet that helps us to focus on burning fat stores and stops us from creating new fat stores in the process.

Metabolism

Metabolism is a misunderstood process.

Many of us love to blame our weight gain on what we call, "our slow metabolism."

Metabolism is actually a very complex process converting what we eat or drink and energy.

The number of calories that our body uses to carry out basic functions is known as our basal metabolic rate. There are several factors that determine what our basal metabolic rate might be including; our body size and composition, our sex, and our age. This basal metabolic rate accounts for almost 70% of our calories burned every day.

In addition to our basal metabolic rate there are other factors that determine the calories we burn each day.

Activities that our body undergoes such as digesting food, absorbing nutrients, transporting and storing food, also takes calories. Our basic physical activity and any exercise we do rounds out our total calorie requirements each day.

Physical activity is one of the most variable factors that determine how many calories we can burn in a day, which is why so many weight loss programs promote it. It makes the program work better and faster.

For our program, we like to use this metabolic process to help us obtain our weight loss goals even without a need for any strenuous exercise.

First, we'll look at the big picture, and then focus on a daily level to better understand how we take advantage of metabolism to achieve our weight loss goals.

An Example We All Can Relate To

Once again, the New Year rolls around and once again we set our New Year's resolution of losing weight.

This year, we are determined to lose weight and get to our goal.

We know a friend who followed a program giving them boxed meals every day, telling them exactly what exercises to do, and our friend lost weight.

We decide this program must be great, and purchase it ourselves.

The first week we enroll and start eating the boxed meals. We follow the exercise program exactly instructed. At the end of the first week we get on a scale and get really excited because we have lost 7lbs! What's the next thing we do?
Our little voice starts talking…

"Seven pounds in seven days, that's a pound a day! That means that in 30 days I will be 30 pounds lighter! I can hardly wait!"

So we start the second week with enthusiasm.

We eat the same meals we ate the first week, even though they really don't seem to taste good. We do the same exercises we did the first week, even though we really don't seem to have the same motivation or energy level. We know we are losing weight, though, so it's all worth it, right? At the end of the second week we get on the scale, expecting another 7lbs or more. What do we see? Only three pounds down!

Now that doesn't make sense, because we did exactly the same thing we did the week before, but we didn't lose the same amount of weight. We are discouraged, but realize we are still losing weight, so the "diet" is working and we're going to stick with it.

That third week is tough.

Same food. Same exercise. Motivation is really lacking now. Then we get on the scale again and can't believe we GAINED a pound! How the heck did that happen, doing the SAME THING we did the first week that caused we to lose seven pounds?

Completely discouraged we stop the program and return to eating just like before.

What you don't understand, though, is this situation makes sense from a medical standpoint.

And here's the reason:

You see; we are designed to survive. What that means is our bodies have survival metabolism, and when it senses something is happening to challenge survival, it responds to correct the suspected problem as best it can.

That first week, your metabolism is humming along at whatever is baseline for our normal activity level. We start our new diet, and guess what? *We are now eating less, maybe exercising more, and so we are burning more calories than we are eating*…and we know what that causes…weight loss.

The first week takes off seven pounds.

The second week, our metabolism realizes something is changing from what it sees as "normal."

 Calorie intake is dropping, so it starts to compensate by slowing down when it can. The second week, we are not burning as many calories, but still more than we are taking in, so we lose some weight.
The second week we lose 3 pounds.

The third week puts our metabolism into a panic.

It realizes that calories coming in have dropped significantly and the demand for energy from any exercise is the same or going up.

The body turns on "survival" mode, slows itself WAY DOWN anytime it can, just to make sure it can bring the calories burned in line with the calories it is getting.

Weight loss stops. We may even gain weight!

Our metabolism will continue to adjust itself to this lower calorie level for as long as we stay there.

The result is a "plateau" in our weight loss requiring us to do one of two things to get over: Lower our calorie intake even more, or exercise more to burn more calories.

Neither sounds much fun to me, and both reasons are typically why individuals drop out of most weight programs.

The time it takes to reach that "leveling out" point may only take a few weeks. Sometimes it takes a few months, but as we know from our own experience, it always shows up if you stay with the same low calories and same level of exercise.

Processing Food Affects Metabolism

Let's use the metaphor of an engine to assist in understanding metabolic function.

Think of your body as an engine, but this engine is special because it runs on three different types of fuel.

Three fuel types that burn differently within the engine. Fast burning sugar, medium burning fats, and slow burning proteins.

The body likes fast burning fuels first. These are easy and quick to convert to energy.

If it can't find a fast burning fuel it looks for medium burning fuels, and if no medium burning fuel is available, it will gladly accept a slow burning fuel.

So the body burns carbohydrates and sugars first anytime they are available, then it uses stored fats, and finally proteins if it must.

Even while sleeping, your body burns energy, usually depleting any carbohydrates first, and then tapping into stored glycogen (we discussed earlier) in the liver. By the time you awaken in the morning your body's engine is idling. It wants to get revved up for the day but it needs some fuel to do that.

It loves to get that fast burning fuel, carbohydrates.

Sugar Is Not Our Friend In The Morning

If you start the day by giving it carbohydrates it will burn through those quickly and start looking for more. This is why typically if you have a high carbohydrate or simple sugar source of energy for breakfast (a biscuit or bowl of sugary cereal for example) you find yourself hungry a few hours later.

If you eat a lot of sugar/carbohydrates first thing and then go sit down at a desk, some of those empty calories get stored as fat for later.

And you still get hungry.

When your body can't find those quick carbohydrates to burn for fuel, it looks for its second favorite source; fat. If there are no carbohydrate available, and no fat stores available, then the body turns to metabolizing protein for energy.

Understanding Protein As An Energy Source

When proteins we eat are digested they are broken down into amino acids so that cells in our body have access to what they need for the job they're trying to complete.

Amino acids help to build muscle, repair bones and skin, and they are also used to produce enzymes which digest foods and help activate our metabolism.

These protein building blocks, amino acids, are very similar to glucose except they contain nitrogen. Because of the nitrogen, amino acids require extra steps to convert to glucose or fatty acids; so they are not the body's first choice or second choice for energy production.

It uses energy to convert protein to usable fuel for the body.

Natural instinct instructs the body to conserve energy, so while protein is an energy source for the body, the extra steps needed for the process and the use of additional energy to convert protein always makes it a last choice when other fuel is available.

We Are All Different

Realize that this short discussion on metabolism is simplified for ease of reading. The processes within the body are extremely complex. While we all use a similar process, each of us has a body with different needs and therefore may follow slightly different paths in utilizing energy.

Marathon and Iron Man competitors do not burn calories like those of us who sit most of the day.

Understanding the basics as outlined in this chapter is enough to help you move ahead with better eating and better weight.

The Struggles We Face With Weight Loss Programs

I know the majority of people reading a book like this are not new to either nutritional studies or the weight loss game.

I bet you're not either, but if this is your first leg a journey into these fascinating subjects, Welcome!

It's no secret there are as many opinions and ideas as there are people involved in this field.

To me, it is important to have either good medically researched data or personal experience to base health decisions on, and although both of those can change over time as well, it makes me feel better to have a firm foundation of relevant and updated information to work from.

What I find is just about all patients and people I work with have the same goals in mind; to lose weight and improve their health.

Most have lost weight in the past is some way or another. Most have tried to adjust their eating habits to improve their nutritional intake.

Making these changes for a "new year's resolution" or for short periods of time when the enthusiasm is high is usually not an issue. The problem for many is being able to maintain healthy eating habits and weight loss for any type of extended period of time.

Some individuals feel for sure there is something medically wrong with them when it comes to losing weight or keeping weight off. They have apparently tried everything under the sun, but never seem to lose weight like everyone else.

They are convinced they will never be able to reach their goal and have all but given up trying.

I don't discount that medical problems do exist, creating issues for some folks.

But experience shows that true medically related weight gain is a very, very small part of the actual population with weight problems.

Regardless of why you are reading this book, I am confident if you follow through you will finish with a renewed sense of strength, knowing you can improve your health and if you desire, your weight issue with the information you gain from this book.

It is also important to point out I work with individuals who may only need to lose 10lbs, and I work with people who need to lose 110lbs or more. I also realize that the 10lbs is just as importance to that individual as the 110lbs is to the other.

The focus of this book does not discriminate, and it does not give specific projections as to how much weight you need to lose. I also cannot make promises to the amount of weight you may lose.

One of the exciting aspects of ideas in the book, is it will work for just about anyone, regardless of your personal eating preferences.

It does not matter if you are a meat eater or vegetarian. It works very well with diabetics. It does not matter how much weight you are trying to lose. I see successful people from all ages and all walks of life.

Your Mind Really Matters

The way we approach eating and weight concerns from a mental viewpoint truly makes a difference to how successful we will be.

I'm amazed that we all have pre-conceived ideas or information we gather from friends and random strangers we like to hold onto as absolute truth, regardless of the qualifications or source.

This hinders our ability to be successful when trying something new.

It may cause us to manipulate this program to fit our ideas and not follow the guidance provided. It can cause us to immediately dismiss something important just because it seems contrary to information we may have come across in our past.

It is important to make clear:

I don't base the ideas or the actions in this book on anecdotal information. I use data derived from medical research or personal experience and results I see from working with actual people who follow the guidelines provided.

If you prefer to take your information from the court of popular opinion or anecdotal information, this book may not be for you.

I want you to feel confident you will successfully meet all the objectives of this program, but if you refuse to let yourself accept new information or open your mind to ideas that may not agree with some past experiences, you should probably not bother to continue reading, and I'm sorry to have wasted your time.

If you are excited about learning something new and helpful, then I'm just as excited to have you continue.

I am absolutely certain your motivation is *the most important part* in determining your success.

A simple point, but sometimes over-looked in the beginning of a weight loss program. A successful and healthy lifestyle requires more than just eating right.

If your mind is not in the right place, you're not ready to really change your eating habits or to lose weight!

Specifically to the idea of weight loss, I want to make a few very important points.

To make this program work for you, it is so important you want this for YOU and not only for someone else.

It is alright to have a goal to impress someone with your appearance, but if you are ONLY trying to lose weight because someone else told you to, your success is limited from the beginning.

Take a few moments to think about why you want to lose weight, and what your personal reasons are for starting this program. Why did you decide to read *this* book?

Consider the two things that are impacted the most with weight loss; Health and appearance.

On the negative side, think about the true dangers of carrying extra weight; early death, increased risk of worsening diabetes and high blood pressure, increased risk of heart and lung disease, increased risk of heart attack or stroke.

On the positive side, think about all the things you would do if you weren't overweight; walk farther, enjoy outdoor activities, sleep better, have much more energy, etc.

Don't Skip This Step!

Now I want you to do something you may not have been asked to do before...write down your goals and dreams concerning your weight loss.

Write down your motivators, your life causes, and the impact of your extra weight.

On the next page is a form you can use to do this exercise.

This is required for your success; to actually use the form provided or a separate piece of paper; *but you must physically write these things down.*

Do you think there is a reason I keep stressing that I want you to actually use a pen or a pencil, a piece of paper, and take the time to hand write these things out?

You can throw them away when you are done if you want, or save them to review during your program. That part doesn't matter, but actually writing them down does!

By going through the motions of actually putting a pen to paper, there is a study that proves you have a greater success rate of meeting your goals, than when you only "think" about your goals or "consider them" and never take the time to write them down[6].

Remember, we all committed to doing things outside our comfort zone and not dismissing things that seemed different when we started, right?

I see difference and results in real-life patients and the statistics proving this point, so I will ask you again...don't skip this section, it is vital to your success.

WRITE DOWN YOUR GOALS--INCREASE YOUR SUCCESS!

I want to lose weight because (ex: for health reasons, appearance, etc):

My personal desire is to weigh __________ and/or get back into a size __________

The last time I remember being at my goal weight or size was when I was _______years old or __________ years ago.

Once I start to lose weight, my desire is to be able to start (walking, exercising, or think of a favorite activity)__? ___ again.

  a. ______________________________________

  b. ______________________________________

  c. ______________________________________

When I get to my goal weight or size, I want to (reward yourself, special activity, change jobs, meet someone, etc. Be specific in what you want to do!) :

  d. ______________________________________

  e. ______________________________________

  f. ______________________________________

What has kept you from being able to lose weight in the past?

What caused you to gain weight in the past (emotions, boredom, stress, lack of self control, poor food choices, didn't know what to eat…etc.)

How are you going to overcome these obstacles as you embark on THIS program?

Weight Loss and Weight Control

OVERVIEW

How am I supposed to eat right to stay healthy and lose weight?

Truth is, it's really not that hard to lose weight once we understand the concept of calorie expenditure.

The problem with most programs is they are not interested in our health, only quick weight loss so we'll be happy and recommend their methods to more people.

Sad to say, but the market only makes money if people need to keep spending it.

They know if they can get us to lose weight quickly we'll feel successful. They also know when we stop their program, the weight will come back and we will go back to them to have the same success again.

It's what's known as a Revolving Door Practice...a great money-making trick too.

 They use drastic or unhealthy methods to get quick results, because quick results are what we all want right?

The downside is any quick weight loss method is not sustainable without significant support and follow-up. We may stick with it for a few weeks, maybe a few months, and then what happens? We go back to eating the same we did before.

Have you ever heard the definition of insanity, "continuing to do the same thing over and over and expecting a different result"?

The weight comes back and then so do you, back to the program that seemed to work so well before. Another big change, liquid diet or all protein meals, or cabbage soup…I think you get the picture.

The more times you cycle your body through this process, the harder it becomes to take the weight off, and the more difficult it is to keep it off.

Why don't we stop this craziness right here, right now?

Think of what you read in this book as a life style CHANGE.

You must commit to changing the way you think about food. You must think about what you eat. You have to stop doing what you are doing and do something DIFFERENT to get new results!

There is a well-known medical fact that makes all weight loss programs work.

It is fairly simple in concept, difficult finding out how to make it work in a way we can tolerate.

I have already mentioned it a number of times; If we burn more calories than we eat, we will lose weight.

Sorry if that doesn't sound like some dramatic revelation.

I know most people are sick of hearing "…. if you would just eat less and exercise more, you would be able to lose weight!"

Me too!

The truth is, I've personally seen a large number of people lose weight just by changing the way they eat, and what they eat, even without exercise.

Don't get me wrong.

Exercise is very important to a healthy lifestyle, but for someone who is significantly overweight, I think it is more important to lose some of that weight first so they can exercise more efficiently.

We also know if weight loss was simple, none of us would have any weigh problems to begin with.

Please remember; our weight loss is tied to a number of different factors that vary for each of us.

It's still true that burning more calories than we eat will cause weight loss, but there are lots of things which influence both of these factors, including genetics, behavior issues, gender, age, and emotions.

For each of us, those items influence our ability to lose weight differently.

The good news is by following the program outlined in this book, we can lose weight regardless of specifically how our body handles any of those things.

I will focus on a process dealing more with using metabolism to take the weight off, regardless of how it is functioning right now.

I know that many of you might say, …"what metabolism?"

Don't worry; this really does work for everyone, and may also help with secondary health issues like type 2 diabetes and high blood pressure.

Let's start by trying to leverage what we know about how our metabolism works.

This about that story I told earlier, when we made our New Year's resolution.

We start to eat a lower calorie diet and we lose weight initially; but after certain amount of time our weight loss seems to plateau.

We are going to combat this by keeping our body from going into the "survival mode" we talked about in that example.

What About When We Eat?

I want to touch briefly on the misconception that eating late is a primary cause of weight gain.

This is not exactly true.

If eating at night was a primary cause for weight gain, then all countries that had problem with people starving would be instructed to feed people at night.

But we don't hear that being recommended, because the issue is more specific.

The problem with nighttime calories is that they tend to be extra calories every time we eat them so they're not burned and stored as fat, i.e., weight gain.

We eat a late dessert. We have a midnight "snack" that sometimes is really an entire meal's worth of food and calories.

The time of day we eat can play an important part as we will see in the program described in this book, but just remember that night time calories need to be included in any calorie count for the entire day.

They can't be ignored or disregarded.

Now, before we discuss setting calorie goals, let's have a strategy planning discussion.

THREE TACTICS TO GET THIS PROGRAM STARTED

Tactic number 1

1. Spend two weeks at a lower calorie intake, followed by one week at a higher calorie intake.

14 days at a lower calorie range, followed 7 days at a higher calorie range. This continued change in calorie intake keeps the metabolism trying to figure out what's going on. We lose weight during the process.

Think about the New Years diet story again.

At the point when your metabolism is thinking it needs to switch to "survival mode" a strange thing happens. IT GETS FED MORE CALORIES. It will respond by turning itself back on, assuming it has no need to slow down.

Just as it gets revved up again, you drop the calorie load, and it has no choice but to burn stored energy…otherwise known as FAT.

As long as you want to lose weight, you keep up this cycle. When you reach your goal, you stop the cycle and the weight loss stops also.

Who would have thought a weight loss program would tell you to eat more food to lose more weight?

When you think about WHY we want to eat more at certain times, it starts to make sense.

It's based on a known metabolic response. It's not magic. The description as to why it works is not vague. You can believe in it, because it is proven to work. In fact, I have seen up to a 30% greater weight loss in patients that use this alternating cycle technique.

Of course, I also had patients that don't believe me.

They start the program and notice after the first few weeks their clothes are loose. Their weight is down, and now they are supposed to eat MORE.

They don't…out of fear of gaining the weight back.

The problem is, they are thinking of the high calorie week as a step back, instead of what it really is, a "fuel the metabolism week".

Without adding the necessary fuel to the metabolic "fire", the fire goes out, and the metabolism slows…. And guess what, they stop losing weight.

All they've done is followed a program just like all the others. Low calorie until the weight loss stops and then comes back.

It usually only takes one time speaking with someone who did the program as recommended, and they realize the need to get back on track.

Daily Food Choices

Drilling down to the daily level, let's talk about what types of food we eat and when we should eat it.

As strange as it may seem, sometimes it's not always what we are eating, but the order our body receives it that makes a difference.

We still must be aware of all the calories we take in, but at certain times of the day, the protein to carbohydrates ratio plays an important part in how our metabolism processes food and determines if it is used as energy or stored as fat.

What I am recommending is a way to get our metabolism to work on energy we have stored as fat, and not giving it other fuel (like carbohydrates) to burn.

It is especially important first thing in the morning or any time after not eating for more than 4 hours. After 4 hours or more, the body has burned through most of its "available" carbohydrates and the metabolism is awaiting its next meal.

We want to start the metabolism back up and start it burning stored fat.

In order to do this, we must start your day with meals that are primarily protein rich.

For those of us who start with a big bowl of cereal, or oatmeal, or a bagel, we will need to start thinking a little differently. Those menu items are nothing but carbohydrates, and our body loves to get a hold of those to burn for fuel.

The other problem with starting the day with carbohydrates is it sets up an insulin response cycle that actually will make us hungrier and cause us to eat more calories than we need a few hours later.

By adding protein to our system at the appropriate time, the body realizes it's time to rev up the metabolism, but it doesn't have the carbohydrates it usually does for fuel, so it looks for the next best thing…stored energy (what we all refer to as FAT!). By eating primarily protein first thing in the morning, the body is forced to use our extra fat as the fuel for the system.

If we wait at least 45min after we eat your protein, you can then add small amounts of carbohydrates to the system without disturbing your fat burning cycle.

The trick to keeping the metabolism going in the direction we want is to continue to use this idea ever 4-5 hours. That means, every 4-5 hours we want to have another protein rich meal or snack. Ideally, this means a <u>minimum</u> of 15-25grams of protein each time with <u>no more than</u> 10grams of total carbohydrates at the same time.

Tactic Number 2

2. Start your day with **at least** 15-25 grams of protein and **less than** 10 grams of complex carbohydrates.

We must program our metabolism to burn the fat we are trying to lose and not provide our metabolism with easy fuel, effectively causing it to ignore stored fat.

No simple sugars or simple carbohydrates first thing in the morning!

No processed breakfast cereals. No orange juice or other naturally or added sugar sweetened beverage.

Many people like oatmeal. Instant oatmeal is bad for our purposes. Unprocessed Oats cooked and not sweetened are not ideal unless you have a high protein shake a hour prior to eating them.

Tactic Number 3

3. Continue to eat 15-25 grams of protein every 5-6hrs throughout the day while awake.

Our goal here is to keep the metabolism working on stored fats, so we continue to provide protein to encourage this activity.

The proteins also require additional baseline energy to breakdown, helping with our fat burning process.

As with any diet that recommends a higher than average protein intake, always discuss this with your healthcare provider if you have any history at all of kidney problems or abnormal kidney function.
This diagram gives you a visual of the way your day should look:

PROTIEN PLACEMENT IS THE KEY TO KEEPING YOUR METABOLISM RUNNING THROUGH THE DAY. IN ORDER TO LOSE WEIGHT, YOU HAVE TO MAKE SURE THAT YOUR FIRST MEAL OF THE DAY IS AT LEAST 15-25gm OF PROTEIN AND NO MORE THAN 10gm OF CARBOHYDRATES.

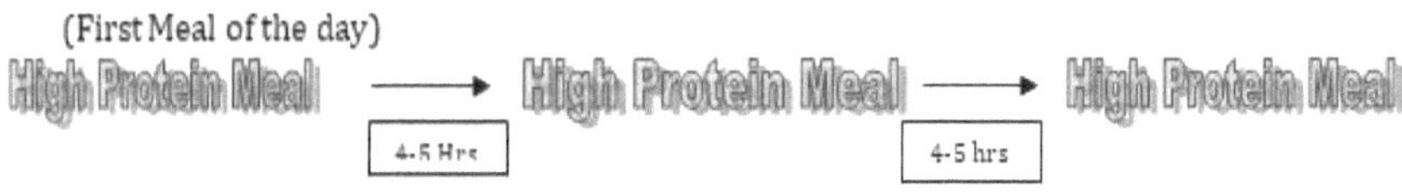

You can eat during the time between your protein heavy times, but you need to wait at least 45min if you are going to add any substantial amount of carbohydrates (more than 10 grams).

Protein placement is very important to keeping your body burning the fat.

This protein placement model, combined with the calorie cycle we talked about earlier are the two KEY issues that will keep your weight loss active.

METABOLISM REVING FAT BURNING CALORIE CYCLE:

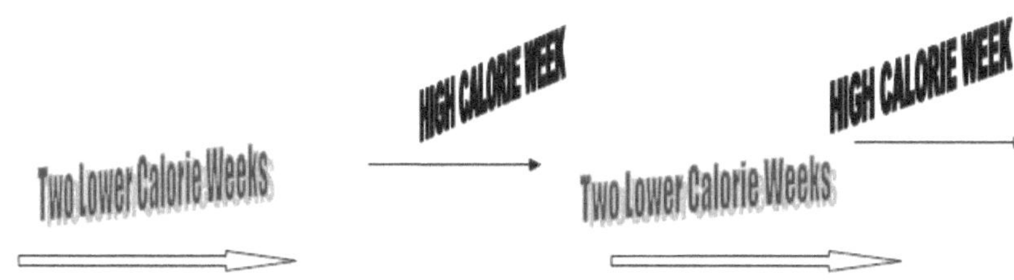

FOURTEEN DAYS ON OUR LOW CALORIE RANGE FOLLOWED BY SEVEN DAYS ON OUR HIGHER CALORIE RANGE AND CONTINUE THE CYCLE FOR AS LONG AS WE WANT TO LOSE WEIGHT

Key Points To Pay Attention To

It is necessary to keep in mind the multiple things affecting how each of us lose weight.

Men will typically lose weight faster than women due to the higher percentage of lean muscle mass, which is a result of genetics (sorry ladies, but I am sure you are aware of this fact).

Because of this, couples using this program should NEVER try to compete or compare results as a way of determining success. It is not a fair comparison.

Likewise, females should not let a factor out of their control discourage them in their weight loss quest.

In addition to gender and other genetic factors, age and behavior also influences weight loss.

How much weight you need to lose can also have a dramatic effect on how fast you will take off the pounds.

If you are close to your healthy weight range and only have a few pounds to lose, you will have to be much more disciplined to get that weight off. Your body will be very sensitive to calorie intake and expenditure. Weight loss is slower. Every time.

On the other hand, if you have 100lbs to lose in order to get to a health weight range, your body WANTS to lose weight.

You will be able to lose more weight initially as you change your eating habits, because your body is already in the weight-loss mode whether you believe it or not. It's just looking for you to give it the right opportunity!

Remember the importance of keeping the protein and carbohydrate timing and balance we discussed earlier.

We talked earlier about your baseline metabolism. This is also know as the Basal Metabolic Rate (BMR), and is basically the number of calories you spend just existing.

To assist with weight loss, our goal is drop down about 500 calories per day below our basal rate to achieve the right amount of weight loss.

You can figure your own baseline if you want to tailor your calorie goals more specifically for you, and your current activity level. Go online and search for "calorie calculators". I have no affiliation with any specific site, but:

Two sites with good information are:
http://www.bmrcalculator.org/ and
http://www.livestrong.com/myplate

Remember weight loss is a *process*.

We did not get to our current weight overnight, and we cannot expect to get to our goal overnight.

I will emphasize again, that there are NO QUICK FIX programs that are truly effective.

If you want to believe there are, or feel the need to continue to try and find one, you don't need to be reading this book.

REVIEW FOR EMPHASIS

Remember, when thinking about calories:

Dietary Fat tends to be stored first and stored fat is utilized for long duration activities first.

- Eat lots of carbohydrates and any dietary fat you eat is bypassed for energy, current body fat is not utilized for energy and additional fat storage takes place
- Eat fewer carbohydrates and once they are depleted, body fat is burned for energy, especially for long duration activities
- Eat _excessive_ fat and fewer carbohydrates and you still will find yourself storing more fat than you are burning and you end up gain weight.

Also, keep in mind why it's harder to lose FAT once you get it:

A Good Reference To Memorize

Calorie breakdown by energy type:

1 g Carbohydrates: 4 calories

1 g Protein: 4 calories

1 g Fat: 9 calories = you have to burn over twice as much energy to lose the same amount of fat than carbohydrates or protein.

Keeping track of Calories

Although no one I ever interact with likes the idea of keeping track of calories, it is imperative that we each get a realistic idea of the number of calories we eat in order to provide a realistic way of adjusting them to get to our goal weight.

On average, all of us tend to under-estimate the number of calories we consume and over-estimate the amount of activity we get each day.

One of the reasons gaining weight is so easy, is due to our tendency to mindlessly put extra calories into our body, fail to pay attention to the number of calorie types in the food we eat, and fool ourselves into thinking that what we eat is healthy when it's not.

Think about it from a logical viewpoint. We gain weight because we eat more calories than we burn.

We need to decrease our calories in order to burn off the fat we have stored as extra weight.

To do this, we really have to get an accurate idea of how many calories we are taking in now that is causing weight gain, right?

Do we have to write down calories for ever? Of course not. But we need to take this step for however long is required to learn the correct amount to eat for our body type.

This step cannot be skipped or this program with fail. I promise.

So I want you to write down everything you eat during the day for as long as you can stand to. I want you to write down the following information every time you put something into your mouth:

Time, Description of the food/drink, total calories, total protein, total carbohydrates

There is a chart in the back of this book to help organize these numbers.

There are also a lot of apps and websites available if you like to use something online.

The Pain Of Counting Calories

Why do I want us to suffer through this process every day? There are a number of reasons, all of which will help each of us get to our goal most effectively.

1. Writing down the food we eat has been shown through scientific studies to cause a greater sustained weight loss than any diet program that does not require this
2. Writing down the food we eat makes us think about what is going into our mouth. We cannot snack without thinking about what we are doing if we have to write things down
3. Writing down the food gives us a visual reminder that helps us stay on track with the requirements of the program.
4. We can see if we are eating the protein we need, at the right time, and balancing the right amount of carbohydrates to make the program work.
5. Our daily diary becomes a tool for weight loss in the future. If we are diligent about writing down what we eat, especially the first month, we will have an "eating guide" to use in the future that we know caused us to lose weight effectively!
6. The only ways to know the actual calories we eat on average every day is to have the information in front of us.
7. When we write down the foods we eat and total the calories every day, we are able to know how much we need to eat on the weekends to raise your calorie levels according to the program goals.
8. If we try and "guess" calorie numbers we will never be as successful as when we actually "know" the right numbers.

A New Way to Count Calories

I do want to make this easier so maybe we can stick with it longer, or at least until we get a better general idea of how many calories we are eating.

So ignore calories that come from protein. Subtract them from the daily calorie totals.

Wait. What did he say?

Ignore calories that come from protein.

Yes protein calories can cause us to gain weight but we also know that protein is the last energy source that our body will go after when looking for fuel.

To our advantage, protein does not cause blood sugar spikes or affect our insulin response, and it can assist with our ability to feel full and not so hungry.

CALORIES THAT COME FROM PROTEIN ARE *FREE* – SO DON'T COUNT THEM IN DAILY TOTALS

This simple fact is one of the great things about this new program. I am not saying this is a fad, "high protein" diet. What I am saying is that when we plan our meals, protein sources allow us to eat more food and still lose weight while watching other types of calories we put into our body.

We are going to focus on being able to look at a food label or look an item up online to find the information you need to keep track of calories.

As you gain experience at this, it will become much easier, and you will start to realize what food you can eat regularly for good health, and what foods you need to limit or even completely stay away from for optimum health and well-being.

All foods with a label shows you total calories, protein, fats and carbohydrates per serving.

We are not counting fat and we are not counting carbohydrates. We are just counting calories and we are only concerned with calories that come from anything but proteins.

We need to always understand the serving size and how much we are going to eat.

For many of us, the serving size on the package is much smaller than what we actually eat, so be sure to take that into consideration.

How To Properly Evaluate A Food Label

When you look at the label on a food product, the unit of measure normally used for protein is GRAMS.

Calories from protein are free; therefore, WE WILL NEED TO CONVERT GRAMS OF PROTEIN TO CALORIES. This is very easy to do!

Each gram of protein produces 4 calories of energy. Look at the product label for the total grams of protein per serving. Multiply this number by 4. This gives us the total calories from protein. Remember, there are 4 calories per gram of protein. THESE CALORIES ARE FREE!

Here is an example:

To figure out the number of calories per serving, we take first take the number of grams (12g in this case) and multiply it by 4 calories per gram, which equals (12 x 4) = 48 calories from protein. We can then subtract that many calories from the total (140 per serving) and end up with 140-48=92 calories per serving. This is the number of calories we count for this particular product.

PRACTICE, PRACTICE, PRACTICE AND SOON YOU WILL BE COUNTING YOUR CALORIE INTAKE WITHOUT EVEN THINKING ABOUT IT.

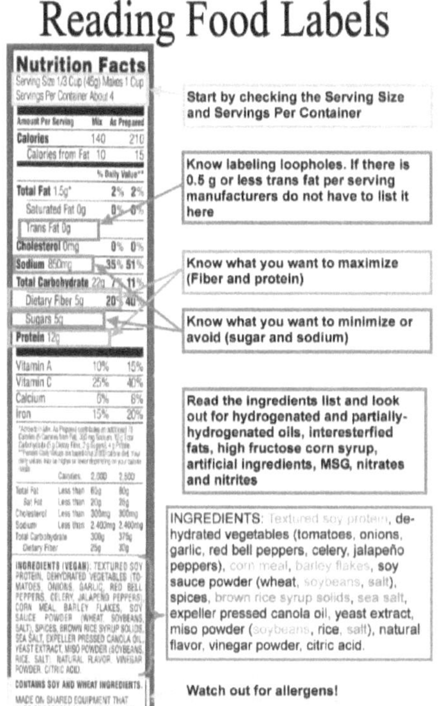

Hidden here is the really good news; but you need to refrain from panic when you see calorie totals.

When counting calories this way, we want to aim for total daily calories that seem much lower than we would imagine.

For women, try and stay with a total around 600-800 a day and for men, around 800-1000 counted calories a day on the low calories weeks, and go up to 200-400 additional counted calories on the high calorie week.

I know these sound low, but the secret is how we count our protein calories, or don't.

We subtract All Protein Calories To Get Our Totals!

Here is an example so you can start to breathe easier about these numbers.

We want to have a chicken breast for dinner, so we use our favorite app or website to find out how many calories and how much protein is in an average chicken breast.

Example from our reference guide:

6 oz chicken breast skinless = 186 calories
Protein = 39 grams

Remember to have a nutritional reference guide available for accuracy and success.

A 170g (6 oz) boneless, skinless chicken breast has about 186 calories.

It also contains about 39 g of protein.

If we do our calculation (39g x 4 calories/g) we find out that 156 calories come from protein, so we don't count those toward our daily totals.

This gives us 186 total calories – 156 protein calories = 30 countable calories.

Written out another way:

39 grams x 4 calories/gram = 156 calories
THESE ARE FREE, SO SUBTRACT FROM THE TOTAL
CALORIES.
Calories you count:
TOTAL calories
186
Subtract Protein calories
-156
Calories added to daily total = 30

30 countable calories for every chicken breast we eat.

We can eat a lot of chicken and still not get to the 600-800 calories we need to count each day!

The same types of benefit come when we eat lean beef, high protein vegetarian sources, or other high protein options.

Higher protein meals can be our friend.

Using this method, we will tend to move away from high sugar or high fat foods, because they contain a lot of calories and we have to count them all.

Using this method will re-train our minds and our eating habits to eat more low fat, low carbohydrate meals and increase our diet of lean proteins and fresh vegetables and fruits.

It's not a high-protein diet. It is a diet that encourages you to eat lower fat and lower carbohydrate meals and increase lean proteins but you work to find a balance that works for your life style.

The program is flexible to who you are.

Even if we are comfortable at 600-800 calories it is very important to increase our calorie intake for 5-7 days the 3rd week then back down again.

This will keep your metabolic momentum at the highest level, which burns up body fat at the fastest rate.

You will find that to get the higher calorie weeks, you get to use those times to eat some of the higher fat and carbohydrate foods you still want to keep in your eating program.

You adjust your life style to an eating program that lets you still have foods you like, but in quantities that are more appropriate for better health.

Always remember the chicken breast example and how protein sources are our best friend when we get hungry. Total Calories = 30!

I think we can agree this makes 600 – 800 calories per day look a lot better and actually attainable.

How many 6 oz. chicken breasts can we eat to get 800 calories at 30 calories each? Very likely a lot more than we are _ever_ going to be able to eat, right?

Fresh green vegetables are not going to add up to a lot of countable calories either

So remember where we will end up getting most of our countable calories:

Three main sources:
1. Starches
2. Sugars
3. Fats
4. Any combination of the above in the form of sauces, dressings, etc.

Some additional information regarding food labels

Paying close attention to what we are eating is so important for improving both our health and our weight.

It is easy to blindly eat whatever we feel like, but not knowing what exactly we are putting into our bodies is counterproductive to maintaining a healthy life style.

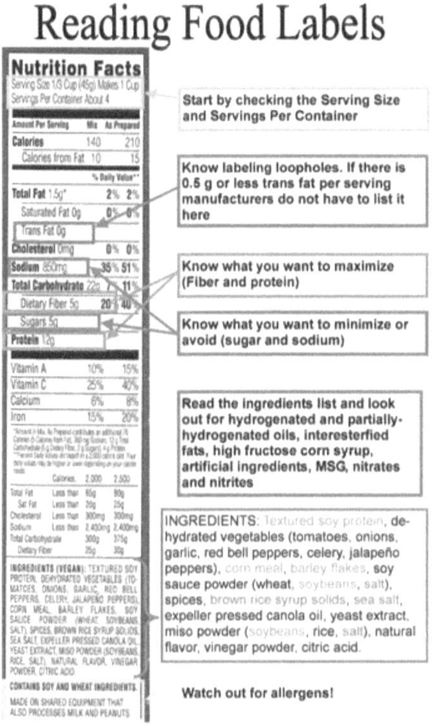

Reading Food Labels

Let's take another brief look at the food label example:

As previously mentioned, always examine the serving size on foods with a label.

For many of us what we are used to eating and what the serving size is for portion control are two entirely different things.

Our normal portion size is typically bigger than the average serving size on packages. We have to be aware of that when counting and keeping track of calories.

Although we are not specifically counting fat calories or carbohydrate calories by themselves (we count total calories in our foods), it's always important to note these on the label and the types of each that are available in what you are eating.

We always want to choose lower fat foods that are higher in fiber content when available. We also want to avoid foods that are high in simple sugars.

Finally, look through the ingredient list. As the box to the left suggests lookout for fats, and sugars that are contrary to healthy options that we understand.

REVIEW THE FIVE BASIC THINGS WE TALKED ABOUT:

To recap the 5 basic things we need to pay attention to for this program to work;

1. COUNTING CALORIES. (Total calories) - (protein X 4) = Calories we count

2. PROTEIN. Our protein intake is time dependent. We need to make sure our protein is greater than carbohydrates first meal of the day and at least every six hours. It is ok to eat protein heavy more often, which is even more effective in boosting your metabolism.   Meet the daily requirement of eating at least 50 - 70 grams of protein per day.

3. INCREASING METABOLISM. Two lower calorie weeks followed by one higher calorie week and repeat the cycle.

4. EXERCISE. Although we did not talk about it yet, exercise will only help with weight loss success and so you should try to get some activity in as you are able. For maximum benefit, activity on 4 out of 7 days for at least 20 - 30 minutes is best. If you are unable to exercise continuously for 20 -30 minutes, it is ok to break up exercise to shorter sessions that you tolerate, just aim to get a total of 20min in the same day.

5. SUPPLEMENTS/LIQUIDS. We will discuss supplements in the next chapter. Drink plenty of fluids as previously discussed.

Any new activity or change takes a little work and effort on your part. Remember to always check with your healthcare provider prior to starting any new eating or exercise program.

It is normal for us to resist change; we want things to stay just as they are or be able take a magic pill and lose weight.

Remember; if you keep doing what you have been doing, you will keep getting the results you have be getting.

You can't keep doing the same thing and expect at some point to suddenly get new results. The laws of nature just don't work that way.

Sorry, but the cold, hard facts are that we *must be willing to change* to reach our goals in life. We do not have to change a lot, just a little and before you know it, you will look back and laugh at your hesitation. Let's face it:

TO LOOK AND FEEL DIFFERENTLY THAN YOU DO TODAY, YOU HAVE TO START THINKING DIFFERENTLY AND APPROACH YOUR EATING HABITS AND LIFESTYLE DIFFERENTLY.

What about alcohol?

The important issue to be aware of when thinking about diets and alcoholic beverages is we know alcohol in any form will slow the metabolism.

People who drink alcohol will have a harder time losing weight than someone who doesn't drink.

If you must drink, it has less of an impact on weight loss if you have a couple of drinks twice a week rather than one or more drinks every night

Alcohol also has empty calories and must be counted. Alcohol is converted to sugar in the bloodstream and so directly affects insulin response.

NUTRITIONAL SUPPLEMENTS

There is controversy regarding whether we need to take nutritional supplements or not.

I am not going to argue either way, but I personally feel that it is important to make sure that we continue to get the proper balance of vitamins and minerals in our diet to stay healthy.

Anytime we change our eating habits, there is a chance we can leave out some important components in our diet. Because of this I believe it is important to add a good nutritional supplement if you have one available.

Finding a good nutritional supplement or multivitamin can sometimes be difficult.

There are a tremendous number of nutritional supplements being bought and sold every day. It is hard sometimes to determine exactly what you do and don't need to take.

There are also other factors to consider which may actually make some of the vitamins you are now taking DANGEROUS. Please read on. If you are truly concerned with your health, you don't want to skip this next part.

A study conducted by the University of Texas in 2004, showed an overall decline in the nutrients found in farmed vegetables due to soil depletion[7].

This infers that even if we eat the healthiest we can every day; we will never be able to get all the nutrition we need from the foods we eat.

Science and medical experts have said this for a number of years. Due to our current trends in farming, the soil no longer supplies the nutrients it did in the past, causing the deficiency we see.

While the government knows this, it won't recommend we take a vitamin or supplement every day for a very specific reason.

Currently ALL vitamin and nutritional supplement companies are regulated at the same level.

They are considered FOOD PRODUCTS and are inspected as such.

To make a law or regulation requiring a higher standard would mean the government would have to start regulating vitamins and supplements and require greater inspections of the manufacturing process.

They can't afford to do that right now (or don't want to due to lobbying pressures!) That's why you see a label on most supplements that states "these statements are not intended to diagnose, treat, or cure and medical conditions" Federal law requires it.

What does that mean to us?

The companies that make the vitamins and any other nutritional supplement you buy off the shelf are held to the same standards as companies that make hot dogs and potato chips!

If understand what the government allows to go into a hot dog and still sell it, you get the picture of how your vitamins and supplements are currently regulated.

It is very disturbing that almost everything you buy at GNC, or Wal-Mart, or your local "Health Food" store also is only required to meet those same standards.

In fact, you could go into business today putting grass clippings into capsules and sell them for whatever you want, and call them whatever you want and the government won't do anything about it. The key is that you are not allowed sell something prohibited, known to cause harm, to make any claims that what you sell has medicinal purposes, cures or prevents disease, etc. Look at the bottles of what you take now, and you will see statements to that same effect.

The guidelines for manufacturing are pretty scary.

A study by an independent consumer-testing laboratory (ConsumerLabs.com) recently highlighted the problem.

They went to a major retail store and bought seven name-brand calcium supplements off the shelf like you or I would. They took them back to their lab and tested them for two things. The first was Bioavailability or the ability of the calcium in the tablet or capsule to actually get into the bloodstream to become useful to the body. The second thing they looked for was the purity of the ingredients; or was there anything in the calcium supplement besides calcium that wasn't advertised on the bottle.

The results were surprising to say the least.

<u>All seven name-brand calcium supplements had a bioavailability of less than 34%!</u>

That means that 66% of what you paid for and took never makes it into your body, and just passes on through.

Even more concerning, however, was the fact that four of the seven *name-brand* calcium supplements had a **detectable lead level** greater than what the FDA considers healthy!

How can this be?

Because the food-grade manufacturing process allows for contamination to take place thing like this are never picked up in "quality control" of food products.

So what Supplements Should I Look For?

The good news is, there are a few companies out there today that really do care about your health, and not just making money selling useless vitamins and supplements.

Only about 1% meets the standards that we recommend – pharmaceutical manufacturing standards (_That means 99% don't meet these standards!_).

These companies manufacture to the same standards as over-the-counter medications such as Tylenol or Advil. They do this voluntarily because there is no requirement to do so, but this commitment to quality assures you that you will only get what you paid for in the supplement, and it will have a bioavailability greater than 95%; so your body will actually be able to use what you are taking.

You have to be careful when you are looking for the right supplement to buy.

There are some companies that throw around important sounding terms like "certified good manufacturing procedures" or Cgmp. Although this means they have some sort of quality control measures, it does not offer any specific guarantee.

Most likely you will not find contaminants in these products, but the bioavailability of the supplements or vitamins may still only be less than 35%. There is no point in spending the money if most of the ingredients just pass through you!

Look for vitamins and supplements that have a few specific things on the labels.

All will have the same disclaimer about medical benefits.

You want to look for "pharmaceutical grade" and also a statement about the bioavailability on the label or in the literature. The USP symbol indicates a high quality manufacturing process. If the company doesn't mention any, they probably don't want you to know how they make them for a good reason.

Don't be fooled by paragraphs from the company saying how good they are if they don't mention specifics about the purity, bioavailability, and manufacturing quality inspection level and back those up with studies, analysis, and a guarantee.

Remember when you are looking at any supplements or other products that claim to help with weight loss, that there are NO MAGIC PILLS. If there were, you wouldn't have to read about it in a big PAID advertisement on TV or in the PAPER. It would be on the news, in medical journals, and talked about all over the world!

The fact of the matter is, there are some supplements that will enhance your weight loss program to a degree, but you still will always have to balance you calorie intake with your calorie expenditure in order to lose weight. That is a scientific fact that cannot be worked around, at least not by any currently known products or procedures.

Read the small print on the bottles or at the bottom of the newspaper ad and TV ad to see the facts about what most companies claim.

They put it in small print, because if it was something they were proud of, or wanted you to really read it, it would be in BIG print and easy to see! Make sense?

PRESCRIPTION WEIGHT LOSS MEDICATIONS

There are prescription weight loss medications available and many can be very effective when used in conjunction with a good eating program.

Some of these medications can be purchased illegally over the Internet.

I don't recommend buying any medications over the Internet for a number of reasons. The number one reason is the concern with safety.

You may have health issues that make these types of medications very dangerous. You may be taking other medications that will interact poorly with Rx appetite suppressants.

Medications bought over the Internet are much more likely to be of a lower quality, and can actually contain things other than what you expect to be getting. There is no way to even be sure that Internet purchased medications were manufactured in the United States. Foreign manufactures may not adhere to the same quality standards as companies in the US.

All these things make the idea of purchasing Internet medication a very unwise choice.

The Real Problem With Rx Weight Loss Medicine

Most people who take medication for weight loss use the medication as the sole aspect of their weight loss program.

Truth is, they can be very effective.

The bad news is, if you depend on them exclusively for your weight loss you will almost certainly gain the weight back as soon as you stop the medication.

I've prescribed them and I know how they work.

I've seen fast initial success but I see more people fail long term when using weight loss medication.

You have to use them in conjunction with a program that modifies your lifestyle and eating habits. The goal of using the medication should only be to help with cravings and portion control.

My advice, if you really feel that you need to use something like Rx medication to assist your program, is to talk to your primary care provider.

They can help you decide what the best choice will be.

Many providers are reluctant to prescribe this type of medication because of the reputation they have for dependence and misuse.

Medical studies also indicate that most patients who use Rx medications will gain the weight back when the medication is stopped. Studies also recommend that medication only be utilized when lifestyle changes and changes in eating habits are ineffective[8].

Anytime I agreed to allow the use of Rx medications with a weight loss program, it was always on a rotation of two months on the medication followed by one month off the medication, with a six month total limit placed ahead of time on the medication use.

This was discussed in depth with my patient and a signed agreement to this schedule was provided for their medical chart.

If you take a copy of this program to your appointment, and let them know you are using the medication as a tool to assist with a structured program, as well as set up a specific timeline with check point goals, they will be much more likely to discuss use of the medication if your medical profile allows you to, but this will always be at the discretion of your personal healthcare provider.

Eating Out

Eating at restaurants and fast food establishments is difficult when changing your eating habits.

The food in any type of restaurant is designed to taste good, so will typically have more fat and more sugars than food you prepare at home.

This is not to say that home food is less tasty, only that the amounts are just about always greater in foods you eat out because it keeps you coming back for more.

Eating out will also have the biggest impact on being successful at losing weight and maintaining weight loss you have accomplished.

A key point to remember is that there is nothing you can do in a single day that will ruin your weight control program.

You can jeopardize your success with certain behaviors if they continue or you make a habit of eating poorly every day; but even if you ate too much of all fattening foods once, you can still recover quickly and get back on track.

You need to maintain the right mental attitude that says, "even if I mess up one day or one meal, it does not give me permission to do it again."

Become determined to pick yourself back up and move in the direction of your goals.

You are strong enough to do this, but have to be mentally willing to make it work.

Tips for success away from home

1. Try to decide what type of food you will order before you get the restaurant. Preplanning is the best defense against poor eating. One of the best resources available online is www.calorieking.com . They have a search feature that will let you get menu items from not only the fast food chains, but also many of the larger franchise restaurants like Appleby's, O'Charley's, Olive Garden, etc. You can plan ahead with figuring the best choices; know the calorie, protein, and carbohydrate components.

2. Try to avoid having bread placed in front of you on the table. You can ask that it be taken off the table if brought traditionally, or at least move it away from your reach. The same goes for chips and other typical complimentary foods. Filler foods that restaurants give away free are always unhealthy for the sake of this program.

3. Avoid foods that are breaded, fried, or covered with sauce. These typically are very high in both carbohydrates and fats.

4. Try to select side dishes that are vegetables instead of starches like pasta or potatoes. If you feel you just have to have a baked potato, get it plain and cut it in half. Season it with lemon, salt, and pepper instead of sour cream, butter, and cheese.

5. If you get a salad, ask for a low calorie dressing, and have it brought on the side. Don't pour it onto your salad. Instead, dip your fork into it before getting each bite of salad. You still get the dressing flavor, but will use much less.

6. Remember, you are the customer paying the bill, so don't be afraid to make special requests that let you enjoy your meal without impacting your new life style! Most eating establishments will be very accommodating if asked politely. They want you to come back.

7. If you frequent a restaurant that always serves large portions, ask for them to provide you with a "to go" container when your meal is brought out and immediately place half of your meal into this container and out of sight. Eat what is on your plate slowly and know you have another meal already set for tomorrow.

More Techniques To Ensure Your Success!

Stay motivated!

You must remember you did not gain the weight in a short period of time, so it would be unhealthy to try and lose it quickly.

You WILL lose weight. You WILL be able to keep it off. You WILL adjust your lifestyle to become a healthier, happier person!

What To Do With Cravings

Give in to them.

I know that sounds counterproductive, but understand why I say this.

Experience teaches if we crave something like chocolate cake and deprive ourselves of it, we tend to eat more of other things that just become additional calories.

Then we end up eating a piece of chocolate cake anyway and feeling guilty about it.

It would be much healthier to have a smaller piece of chocolate cake and get on with it, than to deal with the added calories and mental games when we deprive ourselves of something we really are craving.

 Understandably, this has to be followed with appropriate moderation.

Be Human

Give yourself permission to be human right from the start.

Understand that no one is perfect, and no one can go through this process without stumbling once in a while. It's ok to make a mistake.

What's not ok is to use that mistake as an excuse to make another one.

If you "totally blow it" one day, remember –that is just ONE day – tomorrow is a new day and a new beginning. Your goal will be to get right back on track.

Pick Good Company, Including Yourself

Surround yourself with positive people.

Negative people will make you negative too.

Along the same idea, remember positive "self-talk".

There is a lot to be said for the power of positive thinking. Scientific studies indicate "self-talk" plays an important part in our success day-to-day[9].

If you continually think and speak negatively about yourself, you will be much less successful than someone who works on a positive self-image.

Your ability to lose weight and keep it off is directly related to how you feel about yourself, whether you care to admit it or not. That might be hard to read, but like I said in the beginning, the greatest issue when it comes to weight loss and effectively conquering a weight problem is based on your mental attitude when confronting your problem.

If you think negative things about yourself, you will act in a negative manner.

So, pay attention to your thoughts and make a determination that when negative thoughts creep in, you will replace them with positive ones.

Find a friend or family member who will offer encouragement, but not be judgmental. Let them know from the start what they can do to help or what type of comments you like and what type are not helpful or encouraging.

If they are a true friend, that type of information is what they will want to know.

Write Down Your Goals

And read them often.

Set small goals for yourself and **write them down**, along with a reward when you get to each one.

When you lose 5lbs, treat yourself to something you like to do that doesn't involve eating. Buy yourself a new article of clothing. Go see a movie.

Realize that every journey like this is just a series of small accomplishments, not one big one.

Shortcuts When You Need Them

When you are tired of keeping track or want to give up; make it very easy to stay on track.

When you look at what you are eating, you should always have at least twice as much protein on your plate than anything else.

The next largest portion should be fresh vegetables.

The smallest portion should always be starches or complex carbohydrates, and avoid simple sugars as much as possible.

You have to start your day with primarily protein heavy meal or protein shake.
Try to avoid any carbohydrates first thing in the morning, especially ones high in simple sugars (toast, bagel, waffles, pancakes, etc). That type of breakfast is ok for someone who doesn't have a weight control problem, but you do, so you can't eat like they do.

You can be successful in your quest to lose weight if you approach this with the right attitude. You must focus on changing the way you think about food, and adjust your portions to reasonable amounts.

Remember The Choice Is Always Yours

Some key things to remember as you move ahead include some facts about weight loss and weight control:

1. There is no magic pill or magic solution that requires no work on your part. Think about that logically. With weight control being a big business, don't you think one of the major pharmaceutical companies would spend just about any amount of money to purchase the rights to such an idea? They have BILLIONS of dollars at their disposal for research. Don't believe that a small company has come up with the solution to the world's weight problem; it's just not going to happen. There is no such thing as an easy way out, miracle pill, or "no work" diet. Say that over to yourself a few times and make sure it sinks in. You have to believe that.

2. All weight loss is required to follow the scientific laws of nature. If what someone is trying to sell you doesn't seem logical, it probably isn't. Even if it does seem logical, does it follow known scientific principles or does there seem to be some "magic" involved in the reported outcome? Vague descriptions of a process are usually vague for a reason!

3. You have to be actively involved in the process of weight loss or weight control for it to work. As mentioned before "fix and forget" does not work. Has it ever worked before? If it did, why do you need this book?

4. The world is full of experts. Choose the ones you listen to carefully. Education really does matter more than advice based on "something someone heard sometime…" Your neighbor and your aunt always have good intentions, but always ask for references when someone tries to tell you a "fact" they learned. Sounding like you know what you are talking about and actually knowing what you are talking about through education and experience are two different things. A little knowledge truly is dangerous when it comes to medicine and your health.

And Finally…

It really boils down to making a choice every time you eat.

Do you want to ignore eating the way you know you need to? If you do, then *you are choosing* to be overweight.

If you think about making the right choices, then *you are choosing* to be in control of your weight.

You have to choose to deal with this problem every day.

Choosing takes self-control and discipline. Both of these characteristics are learnable, and will become easier over time.

Saying you have no self-control is a cop-out.

If you really didn't have any self-control, you would have a lot more issues in life to deal with than just weight.

If you want to look for someone or something else to blame (genetics, money, stress, time, etc) then you are actually admitting defeat and are *choosing* to be overweight.

I'm not purposely trying to be mean or uncaring when I say this, in fact, just the opposite. I want you successful!

Sometimes the truth is a hard pill to swallow, but the sooner you make the choice to deal with this every day from now on, the sooner you will start to enjoy life the way you were meant to do!

If reading this last section has made you mad, that's not a bad thing.

Use that emotion to be the basis of your determination to move ahead with your goals.

You can lose weight, and you can keep it off. Tell yourself every night at least three times before you go to bed that you CAN lose weight, and then again three times every morning when you first get up.

- 97 -

YOU WILL SUCCEED!

A Quick Start Option

This is a quick start method for those who absolutely want to lose some weight fast.

It can also be used to jump start your weight loss program.

It is not recommended for everyone, and especially anyone with any underlying health problems such as kidney, liver, or heart disease.

Diabetics should also refrain from following this method.

As with all diet and exercise changes, you must consult with your primary care health provider before starting anything new.

You also need to understand that anytime you make dramatic changes in your eating habits for the sole purpose of losing weight, you have a much greater chance of gaining that weight back plus more if you follow up by returning to the same eating habits you did before.

Rapid weight loss also tends to be fluid loss, which also can be gained back fairly quickly.

With these things in mind, it is important that you only do this rapid weight loss process for no more than 2 weeks at a time, and transition directly into a healthy eating balance to keep the weight from returning and to keep yourself healthy.

The idea for this rapid system is to cut back on your calorie intake, increase your protein intake, and increase your calorie-burning metabolism.

This method follows many other typical high protien, low calorie diet plans because the concepts behind these programs work very well for quick, short term weight loss.

None of these methods are sustainable for extended periods because they are not realistically healthy. They accomplish the goal of rapid weight loss.

You MUST transition to a regular eating program after two weeks regardless of how much weight you've lost or you will jeopardize the effectiveness of the full program described in the this book.

You will not eat regular meals during the day and need to add vitamin and other supplements as indicated to enhance the program in a healthy manner

DAY 1-7

MORNING

First thing you put into your mouth in the morning is a high protein shake.

It must have a minimum of 20grams of protein and no more than 4 grams of carbohydrates.

The bigger the spread between protein and carbohydrates grams the better.

Powdered shakes you mix yourself will allow you to increase your protein more than premixed. You will also take the following supplements:

> 1 Multi-Vitamin
> 1 Supplement with purified white kidney bean (Phaseolus vulgaris) extract
> 500mg of L-glutamine
> ¼ tsp of cinnamon or a 1gm cinnamon capsule

Drink 10-16 oz of water total when taking the supplements.

MID MORNING

Protein bar of your choice that has a minimum of 15grams of protein and TOTAL (not "net or impact") carbohydrates less than or equal to (but not more) than the grams of protein. Drink 10-16 oz of water or a no-calorie liquid without any artificial sweeteners in it.

LUNCH

Protein shake with minimum of 20grams of protein and no more than 8 grams of carbohydrates.

Take the following supplements:
 1 Multi-Vitamin
 1 Supplement with purified white kidney bean (Phaseolus vulgaris) extract

Drink 10-16 oz of water with the supplements

MID AFTERNOON

Protein bar of your choice with a minimum of 20 grams of protein and total carbohydrates equal to or less than the protein grams.
10-16 oz of a no-calorie liquid that does not contain any artificial sweeteners.
A piece of fruit.
 Apple, orange, grapefruit, banana, etc.

DINNER

Protein shake with a minimum of 20 grams of protein and no more than 8 grams of carbohydrates.
Take the following supplements:
 1 Multi-Vitamin
 1 Supplement with purified white kidney bean (Phaseolus vulgaris) extract
 500mg of L-glutamine

Wait 30 minutes. Then eat the following:

Your choice of protein entrée. Baked, BBQ, or Broil without any breading. You can use up to 1 tablespoon of sauce for flavor (ketchup, soy sauce, Italian dressing, etc)
Chicken breast, lean hamburger, steak, turkey breast, lean pork, tofu, etc.

Garden salad with greens, no limit to the size. Option to add celery, cucumber, and a small amount of shredded carrots. No tomatos or croutons.

You can use a small amount of grated cheese if you want.

Do not add dressing to the salad.

Select a Light or low-calorie dressing (less than 80 calories per tablespoon) and put it in a small dish on the side. Dip your fork into the salad dressing before getting a forkful of greens in order to get the dressing flavor on the salad.

No starches, pasta, or breads!

Drink 10-16 oz of water or a no-calorie liquid. Artificial sweeteners are OK with dinner.

EVENING SNACK (if desired)
Select one:
Sugar free jello
Beef jerky
Protein shake
Fruit
Deli meat roll-ups with 2% cheese in them
Low-carb yogurt smoothie (Blue Bunny Carb Freedom are really good)

Drink 8-10 oz of water

YOU CAN REPEAT THIS FOR A SECOND WEEK IF YOU CHOOSE, BUT DON'T STAY ON THIS TYPE OF EATING PROFILE FOR MORE THAN 14 DAYS AT A TIME.

It is imperative that you transition to the low weekday guidelines of the regular program outlined in this book and then follow that program as described.

If you try to use this quick loss program for two weeks, and then return to your normal eating habits, you will usually add too many carbohydrates too quickly. The weight will return plus additional weight, and it will be harder to get it to come off the next time.

REFERENCES

1. Turner-McGrievy, G. M., Wright, J. A., Migneault, J. P., Quintiliani, L., & Friedman, R. H. (2014). The interaction between dietary and life goals: using goal systems theory to explore healthy diet and life goals. *Health Psychology and Behavioral Medicine*, *2*(1), 759–769. http://doi.org/10.1080/21642850.2014.927737

2. Darren C. Greenwood, Diane E. Threapleton, Charlotte E.L. Evans, Christine L.Cleghorn, Camilla Nykjaer, Charlotte Woodhead, Victoria J. Burley. Glycemic Index, Glycemic Load, Carbohydrates, and Type 2 Diabetes. *Diabetes Care Dec* 2013, 36 (12) 4166-4171; **DOI:** 10.2337/dc13-0325

3. Clark, Rober, Frost Chris, Collins Rory, Appleby Paul, Peto Richard. Dietary lipids and blood cholesterol: quantitative meta-analysis of metabolic ward studies. BMJ 1997; 314-112

4. Imamura, F., Micha, R., Wu, J. H. Y., de Oliveira Otto, M. C., Otite, F. O., Abioye, A. I., & Mozaffarian, D. (2016). Effects of Saturated Fat, Polyunsaturated Fat, Monounsaturated Fat, and Carbohydrate on Glucose-Insulin Homeostasis: A Systematic Review and Meta-analysis of Randomised Controlled Feeding Trials. *PLoS Medicine*, *13*(7), e1002087. http://doi.org/10.1371/journal.pmed.1002087

5. Niland, B., & Cash, B. D. (2018). *Health Benefits and Adverse Effects of a Gluten-Free Diet in Non–Celiac Disease Patients*. Gastroenterology & Hepatology, *14*(2), 82–91.

6. Gail Mathews, PhD. Dominican University Study; http://www.goalband.co.uk/uploads/1/0/6/5/10653372/gail_matthews_research_summary.pdf

7. Davis DR, Epp MD, Riordan HD. *Changes in USDA food composition data for 43 garden crops, 1950 to 1999*. J Am Coll Nutr. 2004 Dec;23(6):669-82. PMID: 15637215

8. Michel Erlandson, MD; Laurie C. Ivey, PsyD; and Katie Seikel, DO, RD, *Update on Office-Based Strategies for the Management of Obesity*. Am Fam physician. 2016 Sep 1;94(5):361-368.

9. Tod, David & Hardy, James & Oliver, Emily. (2011). *Effects of Self-Talk: A Systematic Review*. Journal of sport & exercise psychology. 33. 666-87. 10.1123/jsep.33.5.666.

DAILY FOOD AND DRINK DIARY

DATE________________

Range__________________

Daily Calorie

TIME   FOOD/DRINK   CALORIES

PROTEIN   CARBS

LOW CALORIE OR NO CALORIE LIQUIDS: CHECK OFF EACH BOX FOR 6 OZ

TOTAL CALORIES FOR THE DAY _______________ TOTAL PROTEIN __________

Use a new page every day.

Right Food Right Weight

Use your slow metabolism to lose weight

By Bradford Chase, MPAS

* 9 7 8 1 7 2 6 6 7 0 9 4 4 *